REDEFINING VIRILITY: OVERCOMING WEAK ERECTION

A Comprehensive Guide to Reclaiming Your Confidence and Sexual Vitality

ADOOH MARCEL

DEDICATION

This book is dedicated to God almighty and my entire family for their unwavering support, boundless encouragement, and profound love they have showered upon me throughout my life and in the course of writing this book. They are the beating heart of my existence, and I want the world to know just how profoundly appreciate their presence in my journey. And I pray that the almighty God bless them all.

Contents

INTRODUCTION

Erectile dysfunction, often referred to as weak erections or impotence, is a common and often sensitive issue that affects millions of men worldwide. It's important to begin this discussion with an understanding that experiencing weak erections is a normal and prevalent concern that can be caused by a variety of factors, both physical and psychological.

A strong and lasting erection is not only a physical manifestation of a man's sexual health but also plays a significant role in his overall well-being and confidence. When difficulties in achieving or maintaining an erection become persistent, it can have profound effects on a man's self-esteem, relationships, and quality of life.

In this guide, we will explore the multifaceted aspects of weak erections, including their potential causes, symptoms, and the various strategies to address and overcome this issue. Whether you or someone you know is dealing with weak erections, it's important to remember that help and solutions are available, and the road to improvement is often marked with understanding, support, and informed choices.

This guide is designed to provide you with valuable information, practical advice, and resources to help you on your journey to regain confidence and sexual vitality. We will delve into the physical and psychological factors contributing to weak erections, offer guidance on seeking professional help, explore natural remedies and lifestyle changes, discuss medical treatments, and highlight the importance of communication and emotional well-being in the context of sexual health.

As we progress through the chapters, you will find a wealth of information that can empower you to take proactive steps toward addressing weak erections. It's important to recognize that you are not alone in facing this challenge, and there is hope for a fulfilling

Redefining Virility: Overcoming Weak Erection

and satisfying sex life. By gaining a deeper understanding of the issue and exploring the options available, you can take positive steps towards overcoming weak erections and achieving a healthier, happier, and more satisfying life.

Let's embark on this journey together, with the aim of shedding light on a common concern and paving the way for a more confident, vibrant, and fulfilling future.

CHAPTER ONE
DEFINING WEAK ERECTIONS

A weak erection often referred to as erectile dysfunction (ED) o impotence is a condition where a man consistently or recurrentl experiences difficulties in achieving or maintaining an erection tha is firm and long-lasting enough to engage in sexual intercourse o sexual activity. Weak erections can vary in severity, ranging from the inability to achieve an erection at all to having an erection that i not rigid enough for satisfactory sexual performance. This condition can have both physical and psychological causes and may impact a person's self-esteem, relationships, and overall quality of life.

CHARACTERISTICS OF WEAK ERECTIONS

The characteristics of weak erections, often associated with erectile dysfunction (ED), are distinct and can vary in severity from person to person. Here are some key characteristics:

1. **Inadequate Rigidity:** One of the primary characteristics of weak erections is the insufficient rigidity of the penis during an erection The penis may not become firm enough to engage in sexual intercourse or sustain sexual activity.
2. **Consistency or Recurrence:** Weak erections are not just occasional incidents. They occur consistently or recur over time, affecting an individual's ability to achieve a satisfactory erection for sexual activity.
3. **Duration and Sustaining Power:** Weak erections typically lack the necessary duration and sustaining power. Even if an initial erection is achieved, it may not last long enough to complete sexual intercourse, leading to frustration.
4. **Variability:** The degree of weakness can vary. Some individual may experience partial erections, while others may struggle with

maintaining an erection for the entire duration of intercourse. The variability can be influenced by factors like stress or emotional state.

5. **Dependency on Context:** The presence and severity of weak erections may be context-dependent. Psychological factors, such as performance anxiety, stress, or relationship issues, can contribute to the variability in the condition.

6. **Age and Prevalence:** While weak erections are more common in older men, they are not limited to a specific age group. Men of various ages can experience this issue.

7. **Impact on Self-Esteem and Relationships:** Weak erections can have a significant impact on an individual's self-esteem and confidence. They may lead to feelings of inadequacy and frustration. Additionally, weak erections can strain intimate relationships and cause emotional and psychological challenges for both partners.

8. **Distinguishing from Occasional Difficulties:** It's important to differentiate between occasional difficulties in achieving an erection and the chronic nature of weak erections. Occasional issues can happen to anyone and are not necessarily indicative of ED. The consistent or recurrent nature of weak erections sets them apart.

Recognizing and understanding these characteristics is crucial for individuals experiencing weak erections. Seeking appropriate help and solutions, which may include lifestyle changes, medical treatments, or psychological interventions, can lead to improvements in erectile function and overall well-being.

CAUSES OF WEAK ERECTIONS

Weak erections, or erectile dysfunction (ED), can be caused by a variety of physical and psychological factors. Understanding the underlying causes is crucial for effectively addressing and managing the condition. Here are common causes of weak erections:

Redefining Virility: Overcoming Weak Erection

1. PHYSICAL CAUSES:

1.1 Cardiovascular Issues:

- Poor blood flow to the penis is a common cause of weak erections. Conditions like atherosclerosis, high blood pressure, and heart disease can restrict blood flow and impact erectile function.

1.2 Diabetes:

- Diabetes can damage blood vessels and nerves, affecting the body's ability to achieve and maintain an erection.

1.3 Hormonal Imbalance:

- Hormonal imbalances, especially low testosterone levels, can contribute to erectile dysfunction (ED).

1.4 Neurological Conditions:

- Conditions such as multiple sclerosis, Parkinson's disease, and spinal cord injuries can affect the nerve signals that trigger erections.

1.5 Medications and Substance Abuse:

- Some medications, particularly those that affect blood pressure or the central nervous system, can lead to erectile dysfunction (ED). Substance abuse, including alcohol and recreational drugs, can also play a role.

1.6 Pelvic Surgery or Radiation:

- Surgeries or radiation treatments in the pelvic area, often for prostate cancer, can damage nerves and blood vessels associated with erectile function.

2. PSYCHOLOGICAL CAUSES:

2.1 Anxiety and Stress:

- Performance anxiety, everyday stress, and emotional strain can lead to weak erections by interfering with the brain's signals to the penis.

2.2 Depression:

- Depression can reduce sexual desire and affect an individual's ability to achieve or maintain an erection.

2.3 Relationship Issues:

- Problems in a relationship, such as communication difficulties or unresolved conflicts, can lead to performance anxiety and ED.

3. LIFESTYLE FACTORS:

3.1 Poor Diet and Nutrition:

- A diet high in unhealthy fats, processed foods, and low in essential nutrients can contribute to ED. Conversely, a balanced diet can support erectile health.

3.2 Sedentary Lifestyle:

- Lack of physical activity can lead to obesity and poor cardiovascular health, both of which are linked to weak erections.

3.3 Smoking:

- Smoking damages blood vessels and restricts blood flow, making it a significant risk factor for ED.

3.4 Excessive Alcohol Consumption:

- Heavy alcohol use can impair both the physical and psychological aspects of sexual function.

3.5 Lack of Quality Sleep:

- Inadequate sleep can lead to hormonal imbalances and contribute to erectile dysfunction (ED).

Identifying the specific causes of weak erections for an individual may require a medical evaluation. Often, a combination of physical and psychological factors plays a role, and addressing these factors through lifestyle changes, medical treatments, and psychological interventions can lead to improvements in erectile function.

CHAPTER TWO
RECOGNIZING THE SIGNS OF WEAK ERECTION

Recognizing the signs of weak erections or erectile dysfunction (ED) is crucial for early intervention and seeking appropriate help. Here are the common signs and red flags to be aware of:

UNDERSTANDING THE DIFFERENCE BETWEEN NORMAL AND WEAK ERECTIONS

Understanding the difference between normal and weak erections is important, as it can help individuals recognize when they might be experiencing erectile dysfunction (ED) or other sexual health issues. Here's an explanation of this distinction:

NORMAL ERECTIONS:

1. **Spontaneous Occurrence:** Normal erections can occur spontaneously in response to sexual arousal or even during sleep (nocturnal erections). They are not solely dependent on conscious effort or stimulation.
2. **Full Rigidity:** Normal erections are characterized by a full and firm rigidity of the penis, making it suitable for penetration and sexual activity.
3. **Sustaining Power:** A normal erection can be sustained for the duration of sexual intercourse, allowing for a satisfying sexual experience without premature deflation.
4. **Predictable:** Normal erections typically happen predictably when there is sexual desire or arousal. They are not rare occurrences and do not require extraordinary effort.
5. **Consistency:** Normal erections are consistent, meaning they can be achieved repeatedly without difficulty when conditions are conducive to sexual activity.
6. **Minimal Anxiety:** There is usually little to no anxiety or stress associated with achieving and maintaining a normal erection.

WEAK ERECTIONS:

1. **Inconsistent Occurrence:** Weak erections, or ED, involve th consistent or recurrent inability to achieve or maintain an erectio sufficient for sexual activity. They may not occur without medical o psychological intervention.

2. **Lack of Rigidity:** Weak erections lack the necessary rigidity fo penetration and sexual activity, often feeling less firm an substantial.

3. **Limited Sustaining Power:** Weak erections may not last lon enough to complete sexual intercourse. Premature deflation i common.

4. **Unpredictable:** ED can be unpredictable, occurring even when ther is sexual desire, and may not happen when desired.

5. **Inconsistency:** ED is marked by its inconsistent nature. There ma be times when an erection is achieved, but other times when it is not

6. **Emotional Impact:** Weak erections often lead to feelings o frustration, embarrassment, and stress, contributing to performanc anxiety and further exacerbating the issue.

It's essential to note that occasional difficulties with erections ca happen to even healthy individuals due to fatigue, stress, or othe temporary factors. However, when the difficulties become persisten recurrent, or consistently affect one's ability to engage in sexua activity, it's a sign that weak erections or ED may be present. If yo suspect you have ED or experience changes in your erectile functior seeking help from a healthcare provider or specialist in sexual healt is advisable to determine the underlying causes and explor appropriate treatments.

COMMON SYMPTOMS AND RED FLAGS OF WEAK ERECTION

Recognizing common symptoms and red flags of weak erection which are often associated with erectile dysfunction (ED), can hel individuals identify the issue and seek appropriate assistance. Her are the typical symptoms and warning signs to watch for:

Redefining Virility: Overcoming Weak Erection

COMMON SYMPTOMS FOR WEAK ERECTIONS (ED):

1. **Consistent Difficulty Achieving Erection:** The primary symptom of weak erections is the regular or recurrent inability to achieve a sufficiently rigid erection suitable for sexual intercourse.
2. **Reduced Erection Rigidity:** Weak erections are characterized by a lack of full rigidity in the penis. The penis may not become hard enough for penetration or satisfactory sexual activity.
3. **Shortened Duration of Erection:** Weak erections often do not last long enough to engage in sexual intercourse satisfactorily. The erection may subside prematurely during sexual activity.
4. **Inconsistent Performance:** Some individuals with weak erections may experience intermittent or unpredictable erectile difficulties, making it challenging to engage in sexual activity when desired.
5. **Reduced Sexual Desire:** A decrease in sexual desire or libido may accompany weak erections. A lack of interest in sexual activity can be an early sign of ED.
6. **Performance Anxiety:** Worrying about one's ability to achieve or maintain an erection can exacerbate the problem. Performance anxiety can be both a symptom and a contributing factor to weak erections.
7. **Emotional and Psychological Impact:** Weak erections can lead to feelings of frustration, embarrassment, and a decline in self-esteem. A person may avoid or withdraw from sexual activity due to these emotional symptoms.
8. **Relationship Strain:** Weak erections can strain intimate relationships, leading to conflict and frustration between partners. Relationship difficulties can be a significant symptom of ED.

RED FLAGS FOR WEAK ERECTIONS (ED):

1. **Consistency Over Time:** The presence of consistent or recurrent difficulties achieving and maintaining erections is a significant red flag for ED. Occasional difficulties are common and may not indicate a problem.
2. **Medical Conditions:** The presence of underlying medical conditions, such as diabetes, heart disease, or hormonal imbalances,

is a red flag for ED, as these conditions can contribute to erectile difficulties.

3. **Medication Use:** The use of medications that list ED as a side effect should be considered a red flag, as these drugs can affect erectile function.
4. **Age-Related Changes:** While ED can affect men of any age, it becomes more prevalent with age. Experiencing the symptoms of ED and being older is a red flag for the condition.
5. **Relationship Strain:** If there is noticeable strain or conflict in your relationship due to sexual difficulties, it's a red flag that ED may be present and negatively impacting your life.

If you or someone you know is experiencing these symptoms and red flags associated with weak erections, it's advisable to seek professional help from a healthcare provider, urologist, or a specialist in sexual health. Identifying the issue early and exploring appropriate treatment options can lead to improved erectile function and overall well-being.

SELF-ASSESSMENT AND EVALUATION OF WEAK ERECTION

Self-assessment and evaluation of weak erections (erectile dysfunction) can provide valuable insights into the nature and potential causes of the issue. Here's a guide on how to conduct a self-assessment and evaluation:

1. **Frequency and Consistency:**
   - Begin by assessing how often you experience difficulties with achieving or maintaining erections. Are these difficulties occasional, frequent, or consistent over time?
2. **Degree of Weakness:**
   - Consider the degree of weakness in your erections. Are your erections partially rigid but not firm enough for intercourse or are they rarely present at all?
3. **Duration:**

- Evaluate how long your erections typically last during sexual activity. Do they prematurely subside, making it difficult to engage in satisfactory intercourse?

4. **Changes Over Time:**
   - Reflect on whether there have been changes in your erectile function over time. Have you noticed a gradual decline in the quality of your erections?

5. **Spontaneity:**
   - Assess the spontaneity of your erections. Do they occur naturally in response to sexual desire or arousal, or do you require external stimulation or mental effort to achieve an erection?

6. **Emotional Impact:**
   - Consider how weak erections affect your emotional well-being. Do they lead to feelings of frustration, anxiety, embarrassment, or a decline in self-esteem?

7. **Relationship Dynamics:**
   - Examine the impact of weak erections on your intimate relationships. Have there been conflicts or strains in your relationship due to sexual difficulties?

8. **Underlying Medical Conditions:**
   - Review your medical history and any existing medical conditions. Some medical issues, such as diabetes, cardiovascular problems, or hormonal imbalances, can contribute to ED.

9. **Medication and Substance Use:**
   - Take note of any medications you are currently taking and any substances you might be using, such as alcohol or recreational drugs, as these can affect erectile function.

10. **Lifestyle Factors:**
    - Consider your lifestyle, including diet, exercise, sleep, and stress levels. Unhealthy habits and a sedentary lifestyle can contribute to weak erections.

11. **Age and Hormones:**
    - Recognize that age-related changes can affect erectile function. As men age, hormone levels, including testosterone, may decline.

12. **Performance Anxiety:**
    - Reflect on whether performance anxiety plays a role in your erectile difficulties. Are you constantly worrying about your ability to perform sexually?
13. **Quality of Sleep:**
    - Assess your sleep patterns and quality. Poor sleep can lead to hormonal imbalances that affect erectile function.

After conducting this self-assessment and evaluation, it's essential to consult with a healthcare provider or a specialist in sexual health. They can provide a comprehensive evaluation, perform relevant tests, and help identify the specific causes of weak erections. Based on the findings, they can recommend appropriate treatments or interventions to improve your erectile function and overall sexual health.

CHAPTER THREE
SEEKING PROFESSIONAL HELP FOR WEAK ERECTION

Seeking professional help for weak erections (erectile dysfunction) is a crucial step in addressing the issue and finding effective solutions. Here's a guide on how to go about seeking professional help for weak erections:

1. **Choose a Healthcare Provider:**
   - Start by selecting a healthcare provider who can assist with your concerns. You can consult your primary care physician, a urologist (a specialist in male reproductive health), or a specialist in sexual health.
2. **Schedule an Appointment:**
   - Contact the chosen healthcare provider's office to schedule an appointment. Be prepared to discuss your symptoms and concerns openly and honestly during the visit.
3. **Medical History:**
   - During your appointment, your healthcare provider will take a detailed medical history. Be prepared to provide information about your overall health, any existing medical conditions, medications you are taking, and your lifestyle habits.
4. **Symptom Description:**
   - Describe your symptoms of weak erections. Provide details about the frequency, duration, and consistency of your difficulties. Mention any emotional or psychological impact you've experienced.
5. **Underlying Causes:**
   - Work with your healthcare provider to determine the potential underlying causes of your weak erections. This may involve physical examinations and diagnostic tests, such as blood tests to check hormone levels, lipid profiles, and glucose levels.
6. **Psychological Assessment:**

- If psychological factors are suspected, your healthcare provider may refer you to a mental health professional, such as a psychologist or therapist, for a psychological assessment and counseling.

7. **Treatment Options:**
   - Your healthcare provider will discuss treatment options based on the underlying causes and the severity of your weak erections. These options may include lifestyle changes, medication, psychological interventions, or a combination of these.

8. **Prescription Medications:**
   - If prescribed medications (such as phosphodiesterase type 5 inhibitors, e.g., Viagra, Cialis) are recommended, your healthcare provider will explain their usage, potential side effects, and any necessary precautions.

9. **Medical Devices or Procedures:**
   - In some cases, medical devices (e.g., vacuum erection devices) or procedures (e.g., penile injections or implants) may be considered as treatment options. Your healthcare provider will discuss the pros and cons of these approaches.

10. **Follow-Up Appointments:**
    - Regular follow-up appointments may be scheduled to monitor your progress and adjust treatment plans if necessary.

11. **Lifestyle Changes:**
    - Your healthcare provider may recommend lifestyle changes, such as improving diet and exercise habits, quitting smoking, reducing alcohol consumption, and managing stress.

12. **Emotional Support:**
    - Seek emotional support from your healthcare provider or a therapist to address any anxiety, stress, or emotional concerns related to weak erections.

13. **Open Communication:**
    - Maintain open and honest communication with your healthcare provider throughout the process. Share any concerns, questions, or changes in your condition.

Remember that seeking professional help for weak erections is a proactive step toward improving your sexual health and overall well-being. With the guidance of a healthcare provider, you can explore appropriate treatments and interventions to address the issue effectively. It's important to approach the situation with patience, as treatment may take time, and solutions vary from person to person.

THE IMPORTANCE OF CONSULTING A HEALTHCARE PROVIDER

Consulting a healthcare provider when experiencing weak erections (erectile dysfunction) is essential for several reasons:

1. **Accurate Diagnosis:** Healthcare providers are trained to conduct a thorough evaluation, which may include medical history, physical examinations, and diagnostic tests. They can identify the underlying causes of weak erections, whether they are related to physical, psychological, or lifestyle factors.
2. **Rule out Underlying Health Conditions:** Weak erections can be a sign of underlying medical conditions such as diabetes, heart disease, or hormonal imbalances. Healthcare providers can diagnose these conditions and provide appropriate treatment.
3. **Tailored Treatment Plans:** Healthcare providers can create individualized treatment plans based on the specific causes and severity of weak erections. These plans may include lifestyle changes, medication, psychological interventions, or a combination of approaches.
4. **Prescription Medications:** If prescription medications are needed, a healthcare provider can prescribe and monitor their usage. They can also help manage potential side effects and ensure the safety and effectiveness of the medication.
5. **Medical Devices and Procedures:** In cases where medical devices or procedures are required, healthcare providers can explain the options, benefits, and potential risks. They can also perform or oversee such interventions.

6. **Psychological Support:** Healthcare providers can address the emotional and psychological impact of weak erections. They may offer counseling, therapy, or recommend specialists who can help individuals cope with stress, anxiety, or depression related to the condition.

7. **Regular Monitoring:** Regular follow-up appointments with a healthcare provider allow for monitoring of progress and adjustments to treatment plans as needed. This ensures that the chosen interventions remain effective.

8. **Prevention of Complications:** Early intervention through consultation with a healthcare provider can help prevent complications. Untreated weak erections may lead to relationship strain, reduced quality of life, and, in some cases, a decline in overall health.

9. **Education and Guidance:** Healthcare providers can educate individuals about sexual health, lifestyle factors that affect erectile function, and potential risk factors. They can offer guidance on improving overall well-being and sexual health.

10. **Safety and Efficacy:** Consulting a healthcare provider ensures that any recommended treatments are safe and evidence-based. They can help individuals make informed decisions about the most suitable interventions for their specific situation.

11. **Privacy and Confidentiality:** Healthcare providers adhere to strict confidentiality standards, ensuring that personal and sensitive information is kept private. This creates a safe and supportive environment for discussing sexual health concerns.

12. **Empowerment:** Seeking professional help for weak erections empowers individuals to take control of their sexual health. It allows them to explore effective solutions and improve their overall quality of life.

In summary, consulting a healthcare provider is a crucial step in addressing weak erections and related sexual health concerns. It leads to accurate diagnosis, tailored treatment plans, and ongoing support, ultimately improving a person's sexual well-being and overall quality of life. If you or someone you know is experiencing weak erections, don't hesitate to reach out to a healthcare provider.

for guidance and assistance.

PREPARING FOR THE DOCTOR'S VISIT

Preparing for a doctor's visit regarding weak erections (erectile dysfunction) is important to ensure that you get the most out of your appointment and receive the appropriate care. Here are some steps to help you prepare:

1. **Compile Medical History:**
   - Gather information about your medical history, including any pre-existing conditions, surgeries, and current medications. This will help the doctor assess potential underlying causes of your weak erections.
2. **Document Symptoms:**
   - Make a note of the specific symptoms you've experienced, such as the frequency and consistency of weak erections, emotional or psychological effects, and any associated discomfort or pain.
3. **List Medications and Supplements:**
   - Create a list of all the medications, supplements, and vitamins you are currently taking. Include both prescription and over-the-counter drugs.
4. **Record Lifestyle Factors:**
   - Be ready to discuss your lifestyle factors, such as your diet, exercise routine, alcohol consumption, and smoking habits. These factors can impact your erectile function.
5. **Family History:**
   - If relevant, provide information about your family's medical history, especially any history of cardiovascular issues, diabetes, or other conditions related to erectile function.
6. **Psychological Factors:**
   - Reflect on any psychological factors that may be contributing to your weak erections, such as stress, anxiety, depression, or relationship issues. Be prepared to discuss these openly.
7. **Questions for the Doctor:**

- Create a list of questions and concerns you want to address during the appointment. This could include questions about treatment options, potential side effects of medications, and lifestyle changes.

8. **Medical Records and Test Results:**
   - If you have any relevant medical records or test results from previous visits or specialists, bring copies or let your doctor know where they can obtain them.

9. **Prioritization of Concerns:**
   - Prioritize your concerns and questions, focusing on the most pressing issues related to your weak erections. This will ensure that you cover the most important topics during your visit.

10. **Personal Health Goals:**
    - Consider your personal health goals, such as improving your sexual health, overall well-being, or addressing specific lifestyle changes. Discuss these goals with your doctor.

11. **Support:**
    - You may want to bring a trusted friend, family member, or partner to the appointment for emotional support and to help you remember important details discussed during the visit.

12. **Insurance Information:**
    - Have your insurance information ready, including your insurance card, in case it is required during the visit.

13. **Privacy and Comfort:**
    - Understand that the doctor's visit will involve discussing personal and potentially sensitive matters. Be prepared to discuss these issues with the understanding that your doctor is bound by patient confidentiality.

14. **Be Open and Honest:**
    - Finally, remember to be open and honest with your healthcare provider. The more information you provide, the better they can understand your situation and recommend appropriate treatments.

By following these steps and being well-prepared, you can make the most of your doctor's visit, get a thorough evaluation, and work with your healthcare provider to address your weak erections effectively.

MEDICAL EXAMINATIONS AND TESTS

Medical examinations and tests may be conducted to evaluate and diagnose the underlying causes of weak erections (erectile dysfunction). These examinations help healthcare providers identify the specific factors contributing to the issue and determine the most suitable treatment options. Here are some common medical examinations and tests that may be involved:

1. **Physical Examination:** A comprehensive physical examination allows the healthcare provider to assess overall health. They will examine vital signs, including blood pressure and heart rate, and check for signs of cardiovascular issues.
2. **Blood Tests:**
   - **Hormone Levels:** Blood tests can measure hormone levels, including testosterone, to identify hormonal imbalances that might be contributing to weak erections.
   - **Lipid Profile:** High cholesterol levels can impact blood flow, affecting erectile function. A lipid profile can assess cholesterol levels.
   - **Blood Glucose:** High blood sugar levels, as seen in diabetes, can lead to nerve and blood vessel damage, potentially affecting erections.
3. **Psychological Assessment:** A mental health professional may conduct psychological assessments to identify emotional factors contributing to weak erections, such as anxiety, depression, or stress.
4. **Ultrasound:**
   - **Doppler Ultrasound:** This test evaluates blood flow in the arteries of the penis to assess vascular function. It can reveal issues like arterial blockages.
5. **Penile Nerve Function Tests:** These tests assess the sensitivity and function of the nerves in the penis to identify nerve-related causes of weak erections.
6. **Nocturnal Penile Tumescence (NPT) Test:** NPT tests measure spontaneous erections that occur during sleep. An absence of NPT suggests a potential physical cause of weak erections.

7. **Injection Tests:** During a penile injection test, a medication is injected into the penis to induce an erection. This helps determine i the cause of weak erections is primarily physical.

8. **Penile Blood Flow Tests:** These tests assess blood flow in the penile arteries and veins to identify any restrictions or blockages that may contribute to weak erections.

9. **Psychological Questionnaires:** You may be asked to complete psychological questionnaires to assess your emotional state and identify any psychological factors contributing to your condition.

10. **Imaging Studies:** In some cases, imaging studies such as MRI or CT scans may be used to investigate any structural abnormalities in the pelvic region that could be affecting erectile function.

11. **Cardiovascular Assessment:** A thorough assessment of your cardiovascular health may be conducted, as cardiovascular conditions can impact blood flow to the penis.

12. **Metabolic and Hormonal Tests:** Testing for conditions such as diabetes and hormonal imbalances is important, as these factors can contribute to erectile dysfunction.

The specific tests you undergo will depend on your healthcare provider's evaluation of your medical history, symptoms, and suspected causes of weak erections. It's important to be prepared for these tests, as they can provide critical information for an accurate diagnosis and effective treatment plan. Your healthcare provider will discuss the results with you and recommend appropriate treatments or interventions based on the findings.

CHAPTER FOUR
NATURAL REMEDIES AND LIFESTYLE CHANGES

Natural remedies and lifestyle changes can be effective in improving erectile function and addressing weak erections (erectile dysfunction). It's important to note that these approaches may not work for everyone and should be discussed with a healthcare provider. Here are some natural remedies and lifestyle changes that can help:

1. DIETARY MODIFICATIONS:

- **Mediterranean Diet:** Adopt a Mediterranean-style diet rich in fruits, vegetables, whole grains, lean proteins, and healthy fats (olive oil and nuts). This diet is associated with improved cardiovascular health and can positively impact erectile function.
- **Foods for Nitric Oxide:** Include foods high in nitrates, such as beets, spinach, and arugula, as they can promote nitric oxide production, which relaxes blood vessels and enhances blood flow.

2. REGULAR EXERCISE:

- Engage in regular physical activity, including aerobic exercises and strength training. Exercise improves cardiovascular health, enhances blood flow, and can positively impact erectile function.

3. STRESS MANAGEMENT:

- Practice stress-reduction techniques such as meditation, deep breathing exercises, yoga, or progressive muscle relaxation. Reducing stress and anxiety can have a beneficial effect on erectile function.

4. WEIGHT MANAGEMENT:

- Maintain a healthy body weight through a combination of a balanced diet and regular exercise. Weight loss can improve hormonal balance and enhance erectile function.

5. LIMIT ALCOHOL AND SMOKING:

- Reduce alcohol consumption and quit smoking. Both alcohol and smoking can negatively impact blood flow and overall vascular health.

6. SLEEP QUALITY:

- Ensure you get adequate, high-quality sleep. Poor sleep patterns can affect hormone levels and may contribute to weak erections.

7. HYDRATION:

- Stay adequately hydrated, as dehydration can impact blood flow and overall health.

8. LIMIT PROCESSED FOODS:

- Reduce your intake of processed foods, which are often high in salt and unhealthy fats. These can contribute to cardiovascular issues that affect erectile function.

9. HERBAL SUPPLEMENTS:

- Some herbal supplements like ginseng, L-arginine, and DHEA have been suggested as potential remedies for erectile dysfunction. Consult with a healthcare provider before taking any supplements to ensure they are safe and appropriate for your situation.

10. ACUPUNCTURE:

Some individuals have found acupuncture to be beneficial in improving erectile function. Acupuncture can potentially improve blood flow and reduce stress.

11. PELVIC FLOOR EXERCISES:

Kegel exercises, which strengthen the pelvic floor muscles, may help some men improve erectile function and control.

12. COMMUNICATION AND RELATIONSHIP BUILDING:

Open communication with your partner can reduce performance anxiety and improve your relationship, positively impacting your sexual health.

13. LIMIT CYCLING AND PROLONGED SITTING:

Prolonged cycling or sitting may compress nerves and blood vessels related to erectile function. Take breaks and consider using a padded bicycle seat.

It's important to consult with a healthcare provider before making significant changes to your lifestyle or starting any new remedies, especially if you have underlying medical conditions. They can provide guidance, monitor your progress, and ensure that the chosen approaches are safe and appropriate for your situation. Additionally, they can offer further recommendations and interventions if necessary.

CHAPTER FIVE
MEDICATIONS AND MEDICAL TREATMENTS

Medications and medical treatments are common approaches for addressing weak erections (erectile dysfunction). The choice of treatment depends on the underlying causes and individual factors. Here are some of the medications and medical treatments commonly used:

1. ORAL MEDICATIONS (PHOSPHODIESTERASE TYPE 5 INHIBITORS):

These are the most well-known and commonly prescribed medications for erectile dysfunction. Examples include:
- Sildenafil (Viagra)
- Tadalafil (Cialis)
- Vardenafil (Levitra)
- Avanafil (Stendra)

These medications work by increasing blood flow to the penis, helping achieve and maintain an erection when sexually aroused. They are typically taken shortly before sexual activity.

2. TESTOSTERONE REPLACEMENT THERAPY (TRT):

- If low testosterone levels are contributing to erectile dysfunction, testosterone replacement therapy may be recommended. It is administered through gels, injections, patches, or implantable pellets.

3. INTRACAVERNOSAL INJECTIONS:

- Alprostadil is an injectable medication that can be directly injected into the base of the penis. It stimulates blood flow, causing an erection. It is often used when oral medications are ineffective.

4. INTRAURETHRAL MEDICATION:

- Alprostadil can also be administered through a pellet inserted into the urethra, where it is absorbed and helps to induce an erection.

5. VACUUM ERECTION DEVICES (VEDS):

- These medical devices use a vacuum to draw blood into the penis, creating an erection. A constriction ring is then placed at the base of the penis to maintain the erection during intercourse.

6. PENILE IMPLANTS:

Surgical procedures involve implanting devices into the penis. There are two main types:
  - Inflatable implants allow the patient to control when and how long the erection lasts.
  - Semi-rigid implants maintain a constant firmness but can be bent for concealment.

7. SHOCKWAVE THERAPY (LOW-INTENSITY EXTRACORPOREAL SHOCKWAVE THERAPY - LI-ESWT):

- This non-invasive procedure uses low-intensity shockwaves to stimulate blood vessel and nerve regeneration in the penis, potentially improving erectile function.

8. PENILE DOPPLER ULTRASOUND:

- A diagnostic test that evaluates blood flow to the penis. It can identify vascular issues contributing to weak erections.

9. PSYCHOTHERAPY OR COUNSELING:

- For psychological causes of erectile dysfunction, such as performance anxiety or relationship problems, psychotherapy or counseling may be beneficial.

10. SURGERY:

In rare cases, surgical procedures may be recommended to correct vascular or anatomical issues causing weak erections.

The choice of treatment depends on the individual's unique situation and the underlying causes of their erectile dysfunction. A healthcare provider will conduct a thorough evaluation and recommend the most appropriate approach, which may involve a combination of treatments. It's important to consult with a healthcare provider to discuss the benefits, potential risks, and expected outcomes of each treatment option and to make an informed decision based on your specific needs and preferences.

PRESCRIPTION MEDICATIONS

Prescription medications are a common and effective treatment option for addressing weak erections (erectile dysfunction). These medications work by increasing blood flow to the penis, helping to achieve and maintain an erection when sexually aroused. Here are some of the prescription medications commonly prescribed for erectile dysfunction:

1. SILDENAFIL (VIAGRA):

- Sildenafil is one of the most well-known and widely prescribed medications for erectile dysfunction. It is usually taken about 30 minutes to 1 hour before sexual activity. The effects can last for up to 4 to 5 hours.

2. TADALAFIL (CIALIS):

- Tadalafil is known for its longer duration of action, lasting up to 36 hours. This allows for a more extended period of spontaneity in sexual activity. It can be taken as needed or in a lower daily dose for continuous use.

3. VARDENAFIL (LEVITRA):

- Vardenafil is similar to sildenafil in its duration of action, typically up to 4 to 5 hours. It is taken about 30 minutes before sexual activity

4. AVANAFIL (STENDRA):

- Avanafil is a newer medication with a faster onset of action, often within 15 to 30 minutes. It can last for up to 6 hours.

5. LOW-DOSE TADALAFIL (CIALIS DAILY):

- This is a lower-dose formulation of tadalafil that is taken once daily. It is intended for continuous use, allowing for spontaneous sexual activity without planning.

It's essential to use prescription medications for erectile dysfunction under the guidance of a healthcare provider, as they can determine the most suitable medication and dosage based on your specific needs and medical history. They can also provide information on potential side effects and any interactions with other medications you may be taking.

Common side effects of these medications may include headaches, flushing, indigestion, and nasal congestion. Rare but more severe side effects may include vision changes and priapism (a prolonged and painful erection). If you experience any side effects, especially severe or persistent ones, it's important to contact your healthcare provider.

It's worth noting that these medications are not effective without sexual arousal. They do not increase sexual desire, and they should not be used recreationally or without a prescription. Additionally, they may not be suitable for everyone, especially those with certain medical conditions or who are taking specific medications. Therefore, consultation with a healthcare provider is essential to determine if these medications are appropriate and safe for your situation.

MEDICAL DEVICES

Medical devices can be used as a treatment option for addressing weak erections (erectile dysfunction). These devices help improve blood flow to the penis or assist in achieving and maintaining an erection. Here are some common medical devices used in the management of erectile dysfunction:

1. VACUUM ERECTION DEVICE (VED):

- A vacuum erection device is a non-invasive apparatus that uses a vacuum to draw blood into the penis, creating an erection. Once the desired rigidity is achieved, a constriction ring is placed at the base of the penis to maintain the erection during sexual activity. VEDs can be effective for many individuals and have minimal side effects.

2. PENILE IMPLANTS:

- Penile implants, also known as penile prostheses, are surgically implanted devices that are typically reserved for individuals who do not respond to other treatments or who have anatomical issues that prevent them from achieving an erection. There are two main types of penile implants:
    - Inflatable Implants: These implants allow the individual to control the timing and duration of the erection by inflating and deflating the implant with a pump located in the scrotum.
    - Semi-Rigid Implants: These implants maintain a constant, semi-rigid state but can be bent to facilitate concealment when not in use.

3. INTRAURETHRAL SUPPOSITORY SYSTEM:

- Intraurethral suppositories are pellet-shaped medications that are inserted into the urethra using a special applicator. Once in place, the medication is absorbed through the urethral wall, helping to induce an erection.

4. EXTERNAL PENILE SUPPORT DEVICES:

- These devices are designed to support and stabilize the penis during sexual activity, providing additional rigidity. They are typically used in combination with other treatments.

Medical devices are typically considered when other treatment options, such as oral medications, have not been effective or when individuals prefer non-pharmacological solutions. The choice of device depends on the individual's preferences, lifestyle, and the advice of their healthcare provider. It's important to use these devices under the guidance of a healthcare provider or a specialist in sexual health to ensure proper usage and safety.

SURGICAL INTERVENTIONS

Surgical interventions are an option for individuals with weak erections (erectile dysfunction) who do not respond to other treatments or have specific anatomical issues that prevent them from achieving an erection. These surgical procedures aim to improve blood flow to the penis or create an artificial means of achieving and maintaining an erection. Here are some common surgical interventions for erectile dysfunction:

1. PENILE IMPLANTS (PENILE PROSTHESES):

- Penile implants are surgically implanted devices designed to provide a rigid erection when desired. There are two main types of penile implants:
    - **Inflatable Penile Implants:** These devices consist of inflatable cylinders placed inside the penis and a reservoir of fluid located in the abdomen. A pump, typically situated in the scrotum, is used to transfer fluid from the reservoir to the cylinders, creating an erection. When sexual activity is completed, the fluid is returned to the reservoir, deflating the implant.
    - **Semi-Rigid (Malleable) Penile Implants:** These implants maintain a constant, semi-rigid state, allowing the penis to be bent for concealment when not in use.

2. PENILE REVASCULARIZATION:

- In cases where poor blood flow to the penis is the primary cause of erectile dysfunction, penile revascularization may be considered.

This surgical procedure involves redirecting or reattaching arteries to improve blood flow to the penile region.

3. VASCULAR SURGERY:

- In cases where arterial blockages are causing erectile dysfunction, vascular surgery may be performed to bypass or clear these blockages, restoring proper blood flow to the penis.

4. PENILE VENOUS SURGERY:

- For individuals with venous leakage (a condition where blood flows out of the penis too quickly), penile venous surgery can be used to prevent blood from leaving the penis too rapidly, helping maintain an erection.

5. URETHRAL STENT PLACEMENT:

- In cases of venous leakage or other causes of erectile dysfunction, a stent may be placed within the urethra to constrict the blood flow out of the penis, allowing for a sustained erection.

Surgical interventions are typically considered when other treatment options, such as oral medications, vacuum erection devices, or intraurethral suppositories have not been effective, or when anatomical issues are present. These procedures can be highly effective in providing reliable erections, but they also come with potential risks and complications, such as infection or device malfunction.

The choice of surgical intervention and the decision to proceed with surgery should be made in consultation with a healthcare provider or a specialist in sexual health. They can assess the individual's specific situation and provide guidance on the most appropriate surgical approach, taking into account the potential benefits and risks.

CHAPTER SIX
PSYCHOLOGICAL APPROACHES

Psychological approaches are valuable for addressing weak erections (erectile dysfunction) when the condition is primarily related to psychological factors such as performance anxiety, stress, or relationship issues. These approaches aim to identify and manage the emotional and mental aspects contributing to the problem. Here are some common psychological approaches for dealing with erectile dysfunction:

1. COUNSELING AND PSYCHOTHERAPY:

- Individual or couples counseling with a qualified therapist or counselor can help individuals and their partners address emotional issues that may be contributing to weak erections. Therapy can help explore and resolve relationship problems, reduce anxiety, and improve communication about sexual concerns.

2. COGNITIVE-BEHAVIORAL THERAPY (CBT):

- CBT is a goal-oriented and evidence-based therapy that helps individuals identify and change negative thought patterns and behaviors contributing to their erectile dysfunction. It can be particularly effective for addressing performance anxiety and self-esteem issues.

3. SEX THERAPY:

- Sex therapists are trained to address sexual concerns and can help individuals and couples develop healthier attitudes and behaviors related to sex. They can provide strategies and exercises to improve sexual function and satisfaction.

4. MINDFULNESS AND RELAXATION TECHNIQUES:

- Techniques such as mindfulness meditation and progressive muscle relaxation can help reduce stress, anxiety, and performance pressure. These practices encourage individuals to stay present and focused during sexual activity.

5. SENSATE FOCUS:

- Sensate focus is an exercise often used in sex therapy. It involves non-sexual touch and mutual exploration between partners, focusing on physical sensations and emotional connection without the pressure of sexual performance. Over time, this approach can help improve intimacy and sexual function.

6. EDUCATION AND COMMUNICATION:

- Gaining knowledge about sexual health and function, as well as open communication with a partner, can alleviate misunderstandings and create a supportive and stress-free environment for addressing erectile dysfunction.

7. PERFORMANCE ANXIETY MANAGEMENT:

- Techniques for managing performance anxiety, such as relaxation exercises, changing negative thought patterns, and practicing mindfulness, can help individuals regain confidence and reduce anxiety associated with sexual performance.

8. SELF-ESTEEM ENHANCEMENT:

- Addressing issues related to self-esteem and self-worth through therapy or self-help strategies can help improve one's perception of themselves and their ability to engage in satisfying sexual experiences.

9. RELATIONSHIP COUNSELING:

- Weak erections can strain intimate relationships. Relationship counseling can address issues between partners and help restore a healthy and supportive partnership.

It's essential to remember that psychological approaches are most effective when the primary cause of erectile dysfunction is psychological in nature. In cases where there are underlying medical or physical factors contributing to the issue, a combination of psychological and medical treatments may be necessary. Consulting with a qualified therapist, counselor, or sex therapist is an important step in exploring these psychological approaches and finding strategies that work best for your specific situation.

CHAPTER SEVEN
NATURAL AND HERBAL REMEDIES

Natural and herbal remedies are often explored as complementary or alternative approaches for addressing weak erections (erectile dysfunction). While these remedies may offer potential benefits, it's important to approach them with caution and consult with a healthcare provider before use. Here are some natural and herbal remedies that have been suggested for improving erectile function:

1. L-ARGININE:

- L-arginine is an amino acid that the body uses to make nitric oxide, a compound that relaxes blood vessels, helping to improve blood flow to the penis. Some studies suggest that L-arginine supplements may have a positive effect on erectile function.

2. PANAX GINSENG (KOREAN GINSENG):

- Panax ginseng is an herbal remedy that has been traditionally used in Chinese medicine for its potential aphrodisiac properties. Some research suggests it may help improve erectile function.

3. DHEA (DEHYDROEPIANDROSTERONE):

- DHEA is a hormone that is converted into both testosterone and estrogen in the body. Some studies have shown that DHEA supplementation may be effective for some individuals with erectile dysfunction, particularly those with low DHEA levels.

4. PYCNOGENOL (FRENCH MARITIME PINE BARK EXTRACT):

- Pycnogenol is an antioxidant-rich supplement derived from the bark of the French maritime pine tree. Some research suggests it may improve erectile function and overall sexual health.

5. YOHIMBE:

- Yohimbe is an herbal supplement derived from the bark of an African tree. It has been used traditionally as an aphrodisiac. Some individuals have reported improved erections with yohimbe, but it can have side effects and interactions with other medications, so it should be used cautiously.

6. RED GINSENG (PANAX GINSENG):

- Red ginseng is a Korean herbal remedy that may improve erectile function by enhancing blood flow and nitric oxide production.

7. HORNY GOAT WEED (EPIMEDIUM):

- Horny goat weed is an herb used in traditional Chinese medicine for sexual enhancement. Some studies suggest it may help improve erectile function by increasing blood flow to the penis.

8. MACA ROOT:

- Maca is a plant native to the Andes in South America and is believed to have potential benefits for sexual health, including improved libido and erectile function.

9. GINKGO BILOBA:

- Ginkgo biloba is an herbal supplement that may improve blood circulation and has been suggested as a potential remedy for erectile dysfunction.

10. TRIBULUS TERRESTRIS:

Tribulus terrestris is an herbal supplement that has been used to enhance sexual performance and libido.

It's crucial to remember that the effectiveness of natural and herbal remedies for erectile dysfunction varies from person to person. Moreover, the safety and interactions of these remedies with other medications or underlying health conditions should be considered. Always consult with a healthcare provider before trying any natural or herbal remedies to ensure they are safe and appropriate for your specific situation. Additionally, healthcare providers can provide guidance on the correct dosage and potential side effects.

CHAPTER EIGHT
PREVENTIVE MEASURES AND MAINTENANCE

Preventive measures and maintenance strategies can help reduce the risk of developing weak erections (erectile dysfunction) and support overall sexual health. Here are some important steps and habits to consider for preventing and maintaining healthy erectile function:

1. MAINTAIN A HEALTHY LIFESTYLE:

- **Diet:** Adopt a balanced diet rich in fruits, vegetables, whole grains, lean proteins, and healthy fats. A Mediterranean-style diet is associated with improved cardiovascular health, which supports erectile function.
- **Exercise:** Engage in regular physical activity, including both aerobic exercises and strength training. Exercise improves overall cardiovascular health and helps maintain healthy blood flow.
- **Weight Management:** Maintain a healthy body weight, as obesity can contribute to both cardiovascular issues and hormonal imbalances that affect erectile function.
- **Limit Alcohol and Quit Smoking:** Reduce alcohol consumption and quit smoking. Both of these habits can negatively impact blood flow and vascular health.

2. MANAGE STRESS AND ANXIETY:

- Practice stress-reduction techniques such as meditation, deep breathing exercises, progressive muscle relaxation, or mindfulness. Reducing stress and anxiety can have a positive impact on erectile function.

3. ADEQUATE SLEEP:

- Ensure you get enough high-quality sleep. Poor sleep patterns can affect hormone levels and may contribute to erectile dysfunction.

4. STAY HYDRATED:

- Maintain proper hydration, as dehydration can affect blood flow and overall health.

5. LIMIT PROCESSED FOODS:

- Reduce your intake of processed foods, as they are often high in sa
and unhealthy fats that can contribute to cardiovascular issues.

6. REGULAR CHECK-UPS:

- Schedule regular health check-ups with your healthcare provider t
monitor your overall health, manage existing medical condition
and address any potential risk factors.

7. MANAGE CHRONIC CONDITIONS:

- If you have chronic medical conditions such as diabetes, hea
disease, or hypertension, work closely with your healthcare provide
to manage these conditions effectively. Proper management can hel
prevent complications that may impact erectile function.

8. OPEN COMMUNICATION:

- Maintain open communication with your partner about your sexua
health and any concerns related to your relationship. Communicatio
can help reduce stress and anxiety associated with sexua
performance.

9. LIMIT CYCLING AND PROLONGED SITTING:

- Prolonged cycling or sitting can compress nerves and blood vessel
related to erectile function. Take breaks and consider using a padde
bicycle seat.

10. REGULAR SEXUAL ACTIVITY:

Engage in regular sexual activity to maintain sexual function an
support healthy erectile responses.

11. SEEK PROFESSIONAL HELP:

If you notice changes in your erectile function, consult a healthcar
provider promptly. Early intervention and assessment can hel
prevent further issues.

12. MEDICATION REVIEW:

If you are taking medications, consult your healthcare provider t review potential side effects and interactions that may affect erectile function. Adjustments or alternatives may be available.

13. PRACTICE SAFE SEX:

Using protection and practicing safe sex is essential for preventing sexually transmitted infections (STIs) that may impact sexual health.

Taking a proactive approach to your sexual health through preventive measures and maintenance can support overall well-being and reduce the risk of erectile dysfunction. If you encounter any issues or changes in your sexual health, don't hesitate to consult a healthcare provider for guidance and assistance. They can help you maintain healthy erectile function and address any concerns effectively.

CHAPTER NINE
FREQUENTLY ASKED QUESTIONS AND COMMON CONCERNS

Certainly! Here are some frequently asked questions (FAQs) and common concerns related to weak erections (erectile dysfunction) along with answers to provide information and guidance:

QUESTION 1: What is erectile dysfunction (ED), and what causes it?

- **ANSWER:** Erectile dysfunction, or ED, is the inability to achieve or maintain an erection sufficient for sexual intercourse. It can have various causes, including physical factors like cardiovascular disease, diabetes, hormonal imbalances, and lifestyle factors like stress, anxiety, smoking, and excessive alcohol consumption. It can also be a combination of both physical and psychological factors.

QUESTION 2: Is erectile dysfunction (ED), a normal part of aging?

- **ANSWER:** While it is more common as men age, erectile dysfunction is not considered a normal part of aging. Many older men maintain healthy erectile function. ED is often associated with underlying health conditions or lifestyle factors that can be addressed.

QUESTION 3: What are the common symptoms of erectile dysfunction (ED)?

- **ANSWER:** Common symptoms of erectile dysfunction include difficulty achieving or maintaining an erection, reduced sexual desire, and problems with sexual performance. Emotional distress, anxiety, and frustration may also accompany these symptoms.

QUESTION 4: Is it possible to prevent erectile dysfunction (ED)?

- **ANSWER:** While some factors contributing to ED may not be preventable, maintaining a healthy lifestyle, managing chronic conditions, and addressing psychological factors can reduce the risk of developing erectile dysfunction. Regular check-ups and early intervention are key to prevention.

QUESTION 5: When should I see a healthcare provider about erectile dysfunction (ED)?

- **ANSWER:** It's advisable to see a healthcare provider if you experience persistent or recurrent difficulties with erections, as early intervention can be effective. Consult a healthcare provider promptly if ED is accompanied by other concerning symptoms or if it is affecting your emotional well-being or relationship.

QUESTION 6: What should I expect during a medical evaluation for erectile dysfunction (ED)?

- **ANSWER:** During a medical evaluation, a healthcare provider will typically take a medical history, perform a physical examination, and may order blood tests to assess hormone levels and other potential contributing factors. They may also discuss lifestyle and psychological factors that could be relevant.

QUESTION 7: Are there non-prescription treatments for erectile dysfunction (ED)?

- **ANSWER:** Some natural and lifestyle-based approaches can be effective in managing mild cases of ED, but they should be discussed with a healthcare provider. Prescription medications and medical devices are common treatments for more severe cases.

QUESTION8: What are the most common treatments for

erectile dysfunction (ED)?

- **ANSWER:** The most common treatments for ED include prescription medications like sildenafil (Viagra) and tadalafil (Cialis), lifestyle changes, vacuum erection devices, and psychotherapy. In more severe cases, penile implants or surgical interventions may be considered.

QUESTION 9: Can erectile dysfunction (ED) be a sign of an underlying health condition?

- **ANSWER:** Yes, ED can sometimes be a sign of underlying health conditions such as cardiovascular disease, diabetes, or hormonal imbalances. It's important to address these conditions as they can impact overall health.

QUESTION 10: Is it possible to have a satisfying sex life with erectile dysfunction (ED)?

- **ANSWER:** Yes, it is possible to have a satisfying sex life with ED. Many treatment options are available to help individuals achieve and maintain erections, or to improve sexual satisfaction without erections. Open communication with your partner and seeking professional help are essential steps in achieving a fulfilling sex life.

These FAQs and answers provide a starting point for understanding erectile dysfunction and addressing common concerns. It's important to consult with a healthcare provider for personalized advice and treatment options based on your specific situation.

CHAPTER TEN
CONCLUTION

In conclusion, weak erections, or erectile dysfunction (ED), can be a challenging condition, but there are various approaches and solutions available to address it. Understanding the causes, symptoms, and available treatments is essential for individuals seeking to improve their erectile function and overall sexual health.

While each person's journey is unique, the key takeaway is that help is available, and there are numerous effective strategies and treatments to address weak erections. Seeking support, whether from healthcare providers, therapists, or through open communication with partners, is an essential step in improving sexual health and overall well-being.

If you or someone you know is dealing with weak erections, remember that you are not alone, and there is hope for improvement. Consult a healthcare provider to discuss your specific situation and explore the most suitable options for your needs. With the right approach, many individuals can regain their confidence, intimacy, and overall sexual satisfaction.

ENCOURAGEMENT AND MOTIVATION

Facing challenges such as weak erections (erectile dysfunction) can be emotionally and mentally demanding, but it's important to stay encouraged and motivated throughout your journey toward improvement. Here are some words of encouragement and motivation:

1. Seek Support: Remember that you are not alone in facing this challenge. Seek support from healthcare providers, therapists, and your partner. Sharing your experiences and concerns can be a significant source of strength.

2. Persistence Pays Off: Overcoming weak erections may take time and effort, but persistence often leads to progress. Stay committed to your treatment plan and lifestyle changes.

3. Self-Compassion: Be kind to yourself. Recognize that ED is a common issue that can happen to anyone. It doesn't define your worth or masculinity.

4. Explore Options: There are various treatment options available and what works for one person may not work for another. Don't be discouraged if the first treatment doesn't yield immediate results. Keep exploring different approaches with your healthcare provider.

5. Celebrate Small Wins: Celebrate any progress you make, no matter how small it may seem. Each step toward improvement is a victory.

6. Embrace Open Communication: Open and honest communication with your partner is crucial. It can strengthen your relationship and reduce anxiety and pressure related to sexual performance.

7. Stay Positive: Maintain a positive outlook. A positive mindset can have a significant impact on your journey toward improvement.

8. Self-Care: Prioritize self-care, including a healthy diet, regular exercise, and stress-reduction techniques. Taking care of your overall well-being can benefit your sexual health.

9. Embrace Professional Guidance: Don't hesitate to consult healthcare providers, therapists, or counselors. They have the expertise and experience to guide you through your journey to better sexual health.

10. Remember That You Can Improve: Many individuals have successfully overcome or managed ED. Your path to improvement may be different, but with the right approach and support, you can achieve your goals.

11. Take It One Step at a Time: Break your goals into manageable steps. Focus on the immediate steps you can take and trust that they will lead you toward better sexual health.

12. Lean on Loved Ones: Friends and family can provide invaluable emotional support. Don't hesitate to lean on those who care about you.

13. Stay Informed: Knowledge is empowering. Educate yourself about erectile dysfunction, treatment options, and lifestyle changes that can support your journey.

Remember that your journey to improvement is unique, and there is no one-size-fits-all solution. Be patient with yourself, stay determined, and never lose sight of the goal of achieving a satisfying and fulfilling sex life. You have the strength and resources to overcome this challenge.

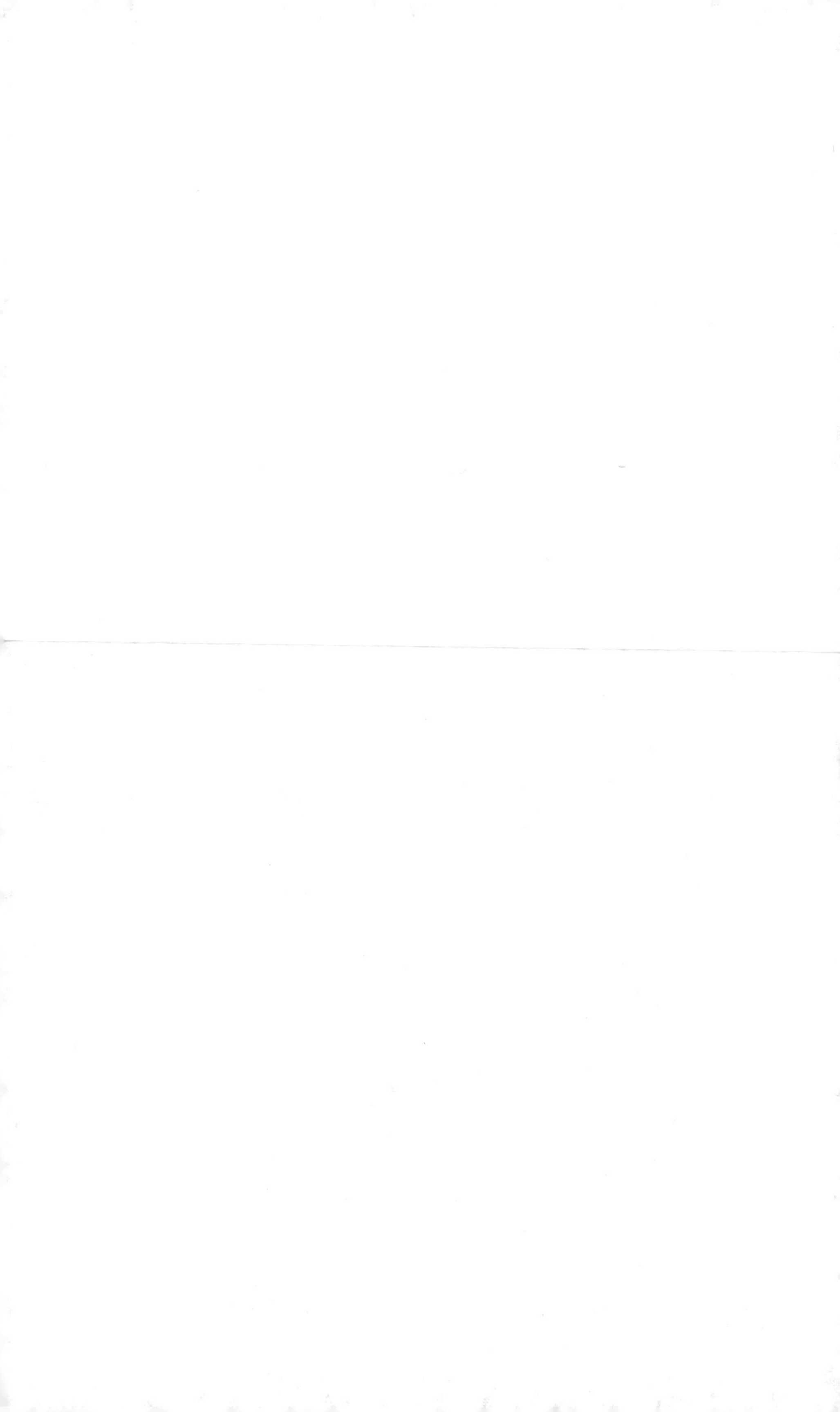

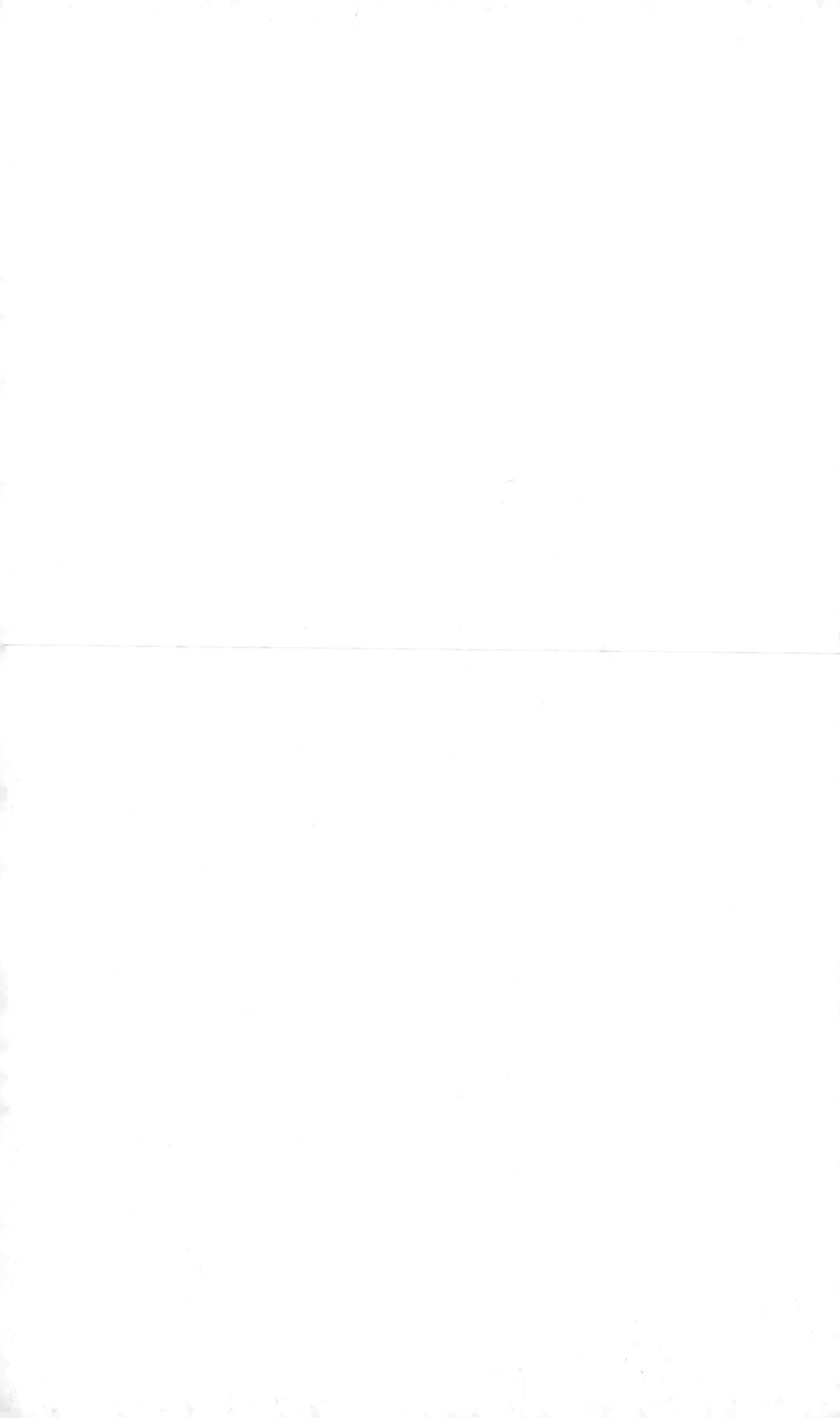